Fast and Effective Exercises for Seniors: 60 Moves to Boost Balance and Mobility

Body Walker

Table of Contents

Introduction

As you get older, you may notice some changes in your balance and mobility. You may feel less stable on your feet, have difficulty walking or climbing stairs, or experience falls or injuries. These changes can affect your quality of life, your independence, and your health.

Balance and mobility are essential for seniors, as they allow you to perform everyday activities and movements, such as standing, sitting, bending, and reaching, lifting, carrying, and walking. They also help you prevent falls, fractures, and other injuries, which can lead to disability, pain, and loss of function. Moreover, they help you maintain your posture, your bone and muscle health, and your cardiovascular health.

The good news is that you can improve your balance and mobility with functional training. Functional training is a type of exercise that mimics everyday activities and movements, such as squatting, lunging, stepping, twisting, and reaching. Functional training helps you strengthen your muscles, bones, and joints, improve your coordination and stability, and enhance your flexibility and range of motion. Functional training also helps you boost your energy, mood, and confidence, and reduce your stress and anxiety.

In this book, you will find 60 fast and effective exercises for seniors that will help you improve your balance and mobility. These exercises are based on functional training principles, and they are designed to suit your level and needs. You can do these exercises at home, at the gym, or anywhere you like, with minimal or no equipment. You can also modify and progress the exercises to make them easier or harder, depending on your goals and abilities.

To use this book and follow the exercises, you will need:
- A comfortable and safe space to exercise, with enough room to move around
- A sturdy chair, a wall, or a railing to hold on to for support, if needed
- A pair of comfortable shoes, preferably with non-slip soles
- A bottle of water to stay hydrated
- A towel to wipe off sweat
- A timer or a stopwatch to keep track of time
- A notebook or a journal to record your progress and feedback

Before you start any exercise, make sure you warm up for at least 10 minutes, to prepare your body and mind for the activity. You can do some gentle stretches, some light cardio, or some mobility drills, to increase your blood flow, heart rate, and body temperature, and to loosen up your muscles and joints.

After you finish any exercise, make sure you cool down for at least 10 minutes, to relax your body and mind and to prevent soreness and injury. You can do some deep breathing, some gentle stretches, or some meditation, to lower your blood pressure, heart rate, and body temperature, and to release any tension or stress.

You can choose any exercise from this book, and do it as often as you like, depending on your schedule and preference. You can also mix and match different exercises, and create your own routines, to add some variety and fun to your workouts. You can also challenge yourself with different equipment, surfaces, and movements, to make your workouts more interesting and effective.

The most important thing is to listen to your body, and do what feels right for you. Don't push yourself too hard, or do anything that causes you pain or discomfort. If you have any medical conditions, injuries, or concerns, consult your doctor before starting any exercise program. If you feel dizzy, nauseous, or unwell during or after any exercise, stop immediately and seek medical attention.

Remember, balance and mobility are not something you **lose** overnight, nor something you **regain** overnight. They are something you can **improve** gradually, with consistent practice and patience. With this book, you will learn 60 fast and effective exercises for seniors that will help you improve your balance and mobility, and enjoy the benefits of functional training. So, what are you waiting for? Let's get started!

Balance and mobility are two essential aspects of physical fitness and health, especially for seniors. Balance is the ability to maintain a stable and upright posture, while mobility is the ability to move freely and easily. Both balance and mobility depend on the coordination and function of various body systems, such as the musculoskeletal, nervous, cardiovascular, and vestibular systems.

Chapter 1
Balance Basics

Achieving balance is akin to mastering the art of maintaining a steady and upright posture, whether you find yourself standing, sitting, or in motion. Picture this: a seamless ability to navigate daily activities like walking, climbing stairs, reaching for objects, or effortlessly rising from bed. Beyond mere movement, balance acts as your steadfast ally in preventing falls, averting injuries, and preserving the cherished gift of independence, particularly vital for our senior community.

Within the pages of this chapter, embark on a journey to unravel the fundamentals of balance, discovering:

1. The intricate body systems and key factors influencing your equilibrium.
2. Practical methods for assessing your balance, unveiling both strengths and areas for improvement.
3. Simple yet impactful exercises tailored to enhance your balance.

4. Techniques for modifying and progressing exercises, adapting them to your unique level and requirements.

5. Insights into seamlessly integrating balance exercises into your daily routine, seamlessly becoming part of your lifestyle.

As you delve into these pages, you'll not only gain a profound understanding of balance but also cultivate the knowledge to enhance it through functional training. This innovative approach mirrors your everyday activities — squatting, lunging, stepping, twisting, reaching — aiming to fortify muscles, bones, and joints, refine coordination and stability, and elevate flexibility and range of motion.

Ready to embark on this transformative journey towards improved balance? Let's take those first steps together!

What is balance and how does it work

Unraveling the Complexity of Balance
In the realm of physical well-being, balance emerges as the silent conductor orchestrating a symphony of stability, whether you find yourself in a standstill, seated, or in motion. Beyond its role in the mundane, balance is the linchpin for daily activities—walking, ascending stairs, reaching for objects, or the simple act of rising from bed. For seniors, it transcends routine; it

becomes a shield against the common and formidable adversaries of falls, injuries, and the erosion of independence.

<u>The Intricate Dance of Body Systems</u>

Balance, though seemingly singular, unfolds as an intricate tapestry woven by diverse body systems and factors. These include:

1. Musculoskeletal System

This foundational system encompasses muscles, bones, and joints, offering the trifecta of strength, stability, and flexibility. It acts as the scaffold, supporting your body weight, cushioning against shocks, and defying the relentless pull of gravity. Furthermore, it grants you the freedom to move your limbs and joints in various directions and ranges.

2. Nervous System

The nerve center controlling voluntary and involuntary movements, the nervous system—comprising the brain, spinal cord, and nerves—directs actions like walking, blinking, and breathing. Simultaneously, it processes sensory inputs from eyes, ears, skin, and organs, sculpting your perception of the environment and adjusting posture and movement accordingly.

3. Vestibular System

Nestled within your inner ear, the vestibular system serves as the sentinel for head position and motion. It collaborates with your eyes and proprioception (the sense of body position and movement) to preserve equilibrium, ensuring you remain steadfast and upright.

Additional Influencing Factors

A myriad of factors, from vision and hearing to medication, nutrition, hydration, sleep, mood, stress, and environment, intricately contribute to or detract from your balance. Quality and quantity play pivotal roles: good vision and hearing bolster awareness, while imbalances in medication, nutrition, and other factors may disrupt the delicate equilibrium.

Balance Unveiled Through Understanding

This intricate dance of body systems and factors illustrates that balance is far from a static trait—it's a dynamic process, continually influenced by a multitude of elements. Armed with this understanding, you're poised to embark on a transformative journey through functional training.

Functional Training: Your Path to Enhanced Balance

Functional training, our beacon in this quest, mirrors the rhythm of daily life—squatting, lunging, stepping, twisting, and reaching. In the chapters ahead, you'll encounter 60 fast and effective exercises curated for seniors. These exercises aren't mere repetitions; they are gateways to strengthened muscles, fortified bones and joints, improved coordination and stability, and an expanded range of motion.

So, with the curtain raised on the intricate ballet of balance, what are you waiting for? Let the journey towards improved balance and mobility commence!

What are the benefits of having good balance

The Multifaceted Rewards of Good Balance

Beyond its role in physical fitness, cultivating good balance becomes a cornerstone not only for bodily health but also for mental and emotional well-being. Unpacking the manifold benefits of possessing excellent balance reveals a tapestry that intertwines physical, mental, and emotional vitality.

✓ **Physical Proficiency and Confidence**

1. Effortless Daily Activities:

- Navigate daily routines with ease—walking, climbing stairs, reaching, or rising from bed—all hinge on the nuanced ability to adjust your body's position and center of gravity. Adequate balance ensures confident execution of these tasks without reliance on external assistance.

2. Prevention of Falls and Injuries:

- Mitigate the risk of falls, fractures, and other injuries, which can significantly impact health and quality of life. Falls, a prevalent concern among seniors, often stem from various factors, with impaired balance being a primary and preventable culprit. Enhancing balance not only reduces the risk but also instills confidence and independence.

3. Posture Maintenance and Overall Health:

- Sustain optimal posture, supporting the alignment of your head, neck, spine, pelvis, and limbs. Good posture distributes body weight evenly, aids organ support, and fends off pain and stiffness. Additionally, bolster bone and muscle health, critical components that tend to diminish with age, safeguarding against conditions like osteoporosis and sarcopenia. A healthy cardiovascular system further ensures vitality, reducing the risk of heart disease and stroke.

✓ **Mental and Emotional Well-Being**

1. Mood Enhancement:

- Elevate your emotional state with balanced exercises that stimulate the production of endorphins, serotonin, and dopamine—neurotransmitters associated with positive emotions. Combat stress, depression, and isolation, common adversaries for seniors, and foster an emotional equilibrium conducive to overall well-being.

2. Cognitive Benefits:

- Engage in exercises that go beyond the physical realm, influencing cognitive processes such as memory, attention, reasoning, and problem-solving. Balance exercises stimulate mental acuity, contributing to cognitive well-being.

3. Social Interaction and Bonding:
- Foster social bonds through improved mobility and confidence. Enhanced balance facilitates better communication and exchange of information, feelings, and support with others, combating feelings of isolation.

✓ **The Gateway to a Holistic Well-Being**
In acknowledging the diverse and extensive benefits, it becomes evident that good balance serves as the linchpin for holistic well-being. The journey toward achieving this balance involves more than mere physical exercises; it delves into the realm of functional training.

What are the common causes and signs of balance problems

Navigating the Complex Landscape of Balance Problems
Balance problems manifest as a disconcerting dance of sensations—unsteadiness, dizziness, and a disorienting feeling akin to the world tilting on its axis. These issues

permeate daily life, impacting routine activities like walking, climbing stairs, reaching for objects, or even the simple act of rising from bed. The ramifications of balance problems extend beyond inconvenience; they escalate the risk of falls, injuries, and a subsequent erosion of independence, heralding severe consequences for health and overall well-being.

Underlying Causes of Balance Problems

1. Inner Ear Disorders:

The vestibular system, a labyrinth of fluid-filled canals and chambers within the inner ear, orchestrates our balance and orientation. Disorders like benign paroxysmal positional vertigo (BPPV), vestibular neuritis, Meniere's disease, and acoustic neuroma can disrupt this delicate system, inducing vertigo—a sensation of movement when stationary.

2. Neurological Conditions:

The intricate network of the brain and nervous system controls voluntary and involuntary movements and processes sensory information. Conditions like stroke, brain injury, multiple sclerosis, Parkinson's disease, cerebellar ataxia, vestibular migraine, and normal pressure hydrocephalus can manifest as balance problems, altering movement and coordination.

3. Medications:

Certain medications, such as antihypertensives, antidepressants, anticonvulsants, sedatives, and opioids, may introduce side effects like drowsiness, dizziness, or low blood pressure. These side effects can compromise coordination, stability, and awareness, heightening the risk of falls.

4. Aging:

Natural aging processes usher in changes—loss of muscle mass, bone density, joint flexibility, and sensory acuity—impacting strength, stability, and mobility. Factors like sarcopenia, osteoporosis, arthritis, cataracts, glaucoma, and presbycusis become potential catalysts for balance problems.

5. Other Factors:

Vision, hearing, nutrition, hydration, sleep, mood, stress, and environmental elements constitute additional influencers. Their interplay, be it positive or negative, dictates the delicate equilibrium of balance. Good vision and hearing act as sentinels against potential hazards, while factors like nutrition, hydration, sleep, mood, and stress can either bolster or disrupt balance and vitality.

Signs and Symptoms of Balance Problems

1. Vertigo:

A sensation of spinning or motion while stationary, accompanied by nausea, vomiting, sweating, and difficulties in walking or standing.

2. Dizziness:

Lightheadedness, faintness, or an unsteady feeling, potentially leading to a feeling of imminent passing out or falling.

3. Loss of Balance or Unsteadiness:

Instability or difficulty maintaining posture or movement, often caused by factors like weakness, pain, stiffness, or sensory impairments.

4. Blurred Vision:

Loss of clarity or sharpness in vision, stemming from eye or brain-related issues, with conditions like cataracts, glaucoma, and macular degeneration contributing to this symptom.

5. Confusion:

Mental disorientation or impaired awareness, with causes ranging from brain-related issues such as dementia or delirium to blood-related problems like low blood sugar or electrolyte imbalance.

<u>Seeking Resolution</u>

1. Prompt Medical Attention:

Given the multifaceted nature of balance problems, any manifestation of the mentioned signs or symptoms warrants immediate medical attention.

2. Diagnosis and Treatment:

A comprehensive assessment by a healthcare professional is essential to identify the root cause of balance problems. Treatment modalities may include medication, surgery, physical therapy, or lifestyle adjustments, each tailored to improve balance, mobility, and avert further complications.

In the intricate realm of balance problems, understanding their origins and manifestations is paramount. Seeking timely medical intervention paves the way for a comprehensive approach to diagnosis, treatment, and ultimately, a restoration of balance and well-being.

How to assess your balance and set your goals

Nurturing Harmony: A Comprehensive Guide to Assessing Balance and Setting Goals

Balance, akin to a symphony of satisfaction, encompasses the diverse facets of life—work, school, family, health, and leisure. Its attainment not only equips you to navigate challenges but also amplifies productivity and overall well-being. However, viewing balance as a fixed destination belies its essence. Instead, it unfolds as a dynamic process, demanding continual adjustment and evaluation.

Steps to Assess Your Balance and Set Goals:

1. Identify Key Life Areas:

   - Utilize a wheel of life diagram to visualize domains pivotal to your well-being—career, education, relationships, personal growth, finances, health, and hobbies. Tailor categories to your preferences.

2. Rate Current Satisfaction Levels:

- Employ a scale of 1 to 10, gauging satisfaction in each life area. Transcribe these ratings onto the wheel of life diagram. Proximity to the center indicates lower satisfaction, while closeness to the edge signifies higher satisfaction.

3. Reflect on Gaps and Imbalances:

- Scrutinize the shape of your life wheel. Is it seamless or irregular? Identify areas of utmost and least satisfaction, understanding their interplay. Acknowledge that discontent in one domain may reverberate across others, forming a holistic perspective.

4. Set SMART Goals for Each Area:

- Embrace SMART criteria—Specific, Measurable, Achievable, Relevant, and Time-bound. Formulate goals with precision. Consider what you want to achieve, how progress will be measured, feasibility, relevance, and set a time frame. For instance, a health-oriented SMART goal could be: "Lose 10 pounds in three months through 30-minute workouts thrice a week and a balanced diet."

5. Create Action Plans and Track Progress:

- Break down each goal into manageable steps, charting them in a daily, weekly, or monthly schedule. Document your action plan, revisit it consistently, and monitor your progress. Acknowledge achievements, celebrate milestones, and adjust your plan in the face of obstacles.

6. Evaluate and Revise Periodically:

- Goals and life priorities are not static. Regularly reassess your goals—every month or quarter. Scrutinize their relevance, realism, and personal significance. Realign goals to evolving circumstances and aspirations. Revisit your wheel of life, gauging any shifts in satisfaction levels and adjust your goals accordingly.

<u>Conclusion</u>

Embark on the journey of assessing balance and setting goals with a systematic approach. Recognize that these endeavors are dynamic processes requiring continual attention and commitment. In this perpetual pursuit of equilibrium, the dividends extend beyond mere achievement—ushering in an elevated quality of life and profound happiness.

15 Balance Exercises

1. Toe Raises
2. Heel-to-Toe Walk
3. Single-Leg Stand
4. Side Leg Lifts
5. Chair Squats

6.   Sit-to-Stand
7.   Step-Ups
8.   Tandem Stance
9.   Flamingo Stand
10.   Clock Reach
11.   Lunge with Twist
12.   Squat with Overhead Reach
13.   Side Lunge with Side Bend
14.   Curtsy Lunge with Arm Sweep
15.   Forward Lunge with Rotation

Elevate Your Balance

Maintaining stability is key to preventing falls and enhancing overall well-being. Engaging in targeted balance exercises contributes not only to better coordination and strength but also reduces the risk of injuries. Here, we delve into 10 comprehensive balance exercises suitable for home or gym settings, requiring minimal or no equipment.

1. Toe Raises

- ✓ **Purpose:** Strengthen lower leg muscles, particularly the tibialis anterior.
- ✓ **Benefits:** Improved balance, flexibility, and prevention of conditions like shin splints and plantar fasciitis.

Execution:

- Sit on a chair, feet flat on the floor.
- Lift toes while keeping heels down.

- Hold for 10s, lower, and repeat 20-30 times.
- Progression: Stand, raise toes, shift weight to heels. Include heel raises.
- Sets: 3 x 10 reps.

2. Heel-to-Toe Walk

- ✓ **Purpose:** Challenge stability by narrowing the base of support, working leg muscles and enhancing posture.
- ✓ **Benefits:** Improved stability, strengthened calves, and enhanced alignment.

Execution:

- Stand with feet together, arms at sides.
- Take a step forward, placing the heel directly in front of the toes.
- Walk for 10-20 steps, maintaining head up and eyes forward.
- Support: Wall or chair if needed.
- Progression: Walk backward, on uneven surfaces, or with closed eyes.

3. Single-Leg Stand

- ✓ **Purpose:** Enhance balance, strengthen core and lower body, and develop ankle stability.
- ✓ **Benefits:** Improved balance, core strength, and reduced risk of ankle sprains.

Execution:

- Stand upright, feet together.

- Lift right foot, balance on left leg.
- Hold for up to 60s, switch legs.
- Support: Chair or wall if needed.
- Progression: Close eyes, move arms or lifted leg, stand on a soft surface.

4. Side Leg Lifts

- ✓ **Purpose:** Target hip abductor muscles for improved stability during weight-bearing activities.
- ✓ **Benefits:** Strengthened hip muscles, toned hips and thighs.

Execution:

- Lie on right side, legs straight and stacked.
- Lift left leg as high as possible without bending the knee.
- Lower leg, repeat 10-15 times, switch sides.
- Progression: Add ankle weights, use a resistance band, or lift both legs.

5. Chair Squats

- ✓ **Purpose:** Strengthen lower body muscles, including glutes, hamstrings, and quadriceps.
- ✓ **Benefits:** Improved posture, alignment, and ease in daily activities.

Execution:

- Stand facing away from a sturdy chair.
- Feet shoulder-width apart, toes forward.

- Bend knees and hips, lowering body towards the chair.
- Gently tap chair, then squeeze glutes to stand.
- Repeat 10-15 times.
- **Easier:** Use a chair with armrests. **Harder:** Use a lower chair, hold dumbbells, or pause at the squat's bottom.

6. Sit-to-Stand

  ✓ **Purpose:** Strengthen lower body and core muscles, enhance mobility and balance, and facilitate daily activities.

Execution:

- Stand in front of a sturdy chair without armrests, feet shoulder-width apart, toes forward.
- Keep spine neutral, head and chest up, engage core.
- Bend knees and hips, lowering body towards the chair.
- Gently tap chair, squeeze glutes and hamstrings to stand.
- Repeat 10 to 15 times.
- **Easier:** Use a chair with armrests, push off for assistance.
- **Harder:** Use a lower chair, hold dumbbells, or pause at the squat's bottom.

7. Step-Ups

✓ **Purpose:** Activate lower body muscle groups, improve balance, coordination, and posture.

Execution:

- Grab dumbbells, stand next to a plyometric box or bench.
- Place one foot on the box, ensuring a 90-degree knee bend.
- Push through the front foot, lift body onto the box, keeping back straight.
- Bring back foot up, tap the box with toe, no weight on it.
- Step down slowly with back foot, return to starting position.
- Repeat 10 to 15 times, then switch legs.
- **Easier:** Use a lower box or bench, or no weight.
- **Harder:** Use a higher box, add more weight, or include a knee lift.

8. Tandem Stance

✓ **Purpose:** Challenge stability, work core and lower back muscles as stabilizers.

Execution:

- Stand upright, feet together, arms at sides.
- Step forward with right foot, placing heel in front of left foot.
- Feet touching or almost touching, head up, eyes forward.

- Hold for up to 60 seconds, switch feet, and repeat.
- Use a wall or chair for support if needed.
- **Harder:** Walk forward/backward, on an uneven surface, or with eyes closed.

9. Flamingo Stand

✓ **Purpose:** Strengthen lower leg, hip, and core muscles, improve balance and flexibility.

Execution:

- Stand upright, feet together, arms at sides.
- Lift right foot, balance on left leg, knee slightly bent, hips level.
- Hold for up to 60 seconds, switch legs, and repeat.
- Use a chair or wall for support if needed.
- **Harder:** Close eyes, move arms or lifted leg, or stand on a soft surface.

10. Clock Reach

✓ **Purpose:** Improve balance, coordination, and strength in lower body, core, and shoulders.

Execution:

- Stand upright, feet together, arms at sides.
- Imagine standing in the center of a clock, hold the chair with left hand.
- Lift right leg, extend right arm to "12", then "3", "6", "3", and back to "12".

- Repeat 10 to 15 times, then switch legs and arms.
- **Easier:** Use two chairs for support.
- **Harder:** Do it without holding the chair, with eyes closed, or on an unstable surface.

Explanation of the 12, 3, 6 position

The "12, 3, 6 position" refers to specific points on an imaginary clock face, and during the Clock Reach exercise, it dictates the direction in which you extend your arm. Here's a detailed breakdown:

1. "12" Position:
- ✓ Stand with your feet together, holding the chair with your left hand.
- ✓ Lift your right leg off the ground.
- ✓ Extend your right arm straight in front of you, pointing toward the imaginary "12" on the clock face. Your arm should be aligned with your shoulder.

2. "3" Position:
- ✓ While maintaining balance on your left leg, smoothly move your right arm to the side, pointing toward the imaginary "3" on the clock face. Your arm should be parallel to the ground.

3. "6" Position:

- ✓ Continuing the sequence, reach your right arm behind you, pointing toward the imaginary "6" on the clock face. Your arm should move backward while keeping it straight.

The "6 position" refers to the direction in which you extend your arm, similar to the hours on a clock face.
"6" Position:
- ✓ Stand upright with your feet together, facing forward.
- ✓ Imagine an imaginary clock beneath you, with the number "6" directly behind you.
- ✓ While maintaining balance on one leg (let's say your left leg for clarity):
- ✓ Extend your right arm backward, pointing toward the imaginary "6" on the clock face.
- ✓ Your arm should move straight back behind you, in line with your shoulder and parallel to the ground.
- ✓ Simultaneously, your right leg, which is lifted off the ground, may extend slightly backward for counterbalance.
- ✓ This movement challenges your balance, engages your core, and activates muscles in your lower back, glutes, and hamstrings.

Visualizing the clock face helps guide the direction of your arm movement during the exercise. The "6 position" involves reaching backward, and its one part of the Clock Reach sequence that aims to enhance your balance, coordination, and muscle strength.

4. Returning to "3" Position:
- ✓ Bring your arm back to the side, pointing toward the imaginary "3" on the clock face. Again, your arm should be parallel to the ground.

5. Returning to "12" Position:
- ✓ Finally, bring your arm back to the front, pointing toward the imaginary "12" on the clock face. This completes one full repetition of the sequence.

During this entire movement, it's crucial to maintain a straight posture, engage your core muscles, and control the motion. The Clock Reach exercise enhances coordination, challenges your stability, and works on the strength of various muscle groups in your lower body, core, and shoulders.

11. Lunge with Twist
- Start by standing with your feet hip-width apart.
- Take a step forward with your right foot into a lunge position.
- As you lunge, rotate your torso to the right, bringing your hands together.

- Return to the starting position and switch to the left leg.
- This exercise engages your lower body, enhances stability, and challenges your core muscles.

12. Squat with Overhead Reach
- Stand with your feet shoulder-width apart.
- Perform a squat by bending your knees and lowering your hips.
- As you return to the standing position, lift your arms overhead.
- This combines lower body strength with an upper body stretch, improving overall balance.

13. Side Lunge with Side Bend
- Stand with feet together, hands on your hips.
- Take a step to the right, bending your right knee while keeping the left leg straight.
- Simultaneously, bend your upper body to the right, bringing your right hand toward the floor.
- Return to the starting position and switch to the left side.
- This exercise targets the inner and outer thighs, improving lateral stability.

14. Curtsy Lunge with Arm Sweep
- Begin by standing with your feet hip-width apart.

- Step your left foot diagonally behind your right leg, bending both knees.
- As you lunge, sweep your left arm across your body, reaching toward the right.
- Return to the starting position and switch to the other side.
- This exercise challenges balance and engages the muscles in your legs and core.

15. Forward Lunge with Rotation
- Stand with feet hip-width apart.
- Step forward with your right foot into a lunge, lowering your hips.
- Rotate your torso to the right, keeping your core engaged.
- Return to the starting position and switch to the left leg.
- The combination of lunging and rotation enhances balance and works your core muscles.

Remember to start with exercises that match your current fitness level, gradually progressing to more challenging variations as your balance improves. Always prioritize proper form and control during each movement.

Chapter 2

Mobility matters

Your ability to move freely is a cornerstone of a vibrant and independent life. However, factors like aging, injuries, or health conditions can impact mobility, affecting your overall well-being. In this chapter, delve into the significance of mobility, unravel why it's pivotal, and explore practical exercises and lifestyle adjustments to boost it. Uncover the holistic advantages of improved mobility on your physical, mental, and emotional health. Equip yourself with the insights and guidance here to preserve or elevate your mobility, paving the way for a more dynamic and satisfying lifestyle.

What is mobility and how does it work

Exploring Mobility: A Holistic Approach to Movement

Mobility, the seamless ability to move your body across diverse situations, is a cornerstone of health and independence. This intricate coordination involves your muscles, joints, nerves, and brain working in harmony, resulting in smooth and efficient movements that impact various aspects of your life.

At its core, mobility integrates three pivotal components: flexibility, strength, and balance. Flexibility encompasses the range of motion in your joints and the elasticity of muscles and connective tissues. Strength represents the force your muscles can generate to propel joint movement and support your body. Balance, meanwhile, focuses on maintaining posture and stability during movement or stillness. Together, these components enable you to navigate your body through different dimensions, speeds, and complexities.

Elevating your mobility involves a consistent commitment to enhancing all three components. Incorporating diverse exercises and activities becomes crucial in challenging your flexibility, strength, and balance. Engage in practices like stretching, yoga, or pilates to amplify flexibility, leverage resistance training, bodyweight exercises, or functional movements for strength, and embrace activities such as tai chi, dance, or specialized balance exercises to refine your stability. Integrate mobility drills like joint rotations, dynamic stretches, and locomotion patterns into your routine to prepare your body for movement.

The benefits of cultivating mobility are far-reaching, including:

- Alleviation of pain and stiffness in joints and muscles
- Improvement in posture and alignment, benefitting the spine and limbs
- Expansion of your range of motion, fostering fluidity in movements
- Amplification of performance and efficiency in sports and physical activities
- Reduction in the risk of falls and injuries
- Enhancement of blood circulation and oxygen delivery to tissues
- Upliftment of mood and mental well-being

Understanding the intricacies of mobility empowers you to proactively improve it, paving the way for a more active, enriching, and fulfilling life.

What are the benefits of having good mobility

Unlocking the Power of Mobility: A Comprehensive Guide

Achieving optimal mobility signifies the ability to move your body effortlessly across diverse scenarios and environments. This intricate process involves the seamless coordination of muscles, joints, nerves, and the brain, resulting in fluid and efficient movements.

The significance of good mobility extends beyond the physical realm, impacting your overall health, well-being, and independence by facilitating daily activities, preventing injuries, and enhancing your quality of life.

Let's delve into the multifaceted benefits that accompany the cultivation of good mobility:

1. Reduced Pain and Stiffness:
- Good mobility plays a pivotal role in preventing or alleviating conditions such as arthritis, osteoporosis, and fibromyalgia.
- Regular movement lubricates joints, increases blood flow, and mitigates inflammation and tension.

2. Improved Posture and Alignment:
- Maintaining proper posture and alignment becomes achievable with good mobility, preventing or addressing issues like back pain, neck pain, and headaches.
- A neutral position of the spine and limbs minimizes stress on muscles, ligaments, and discs.

3. Increased Range of Motion:
- Good mobility empowers you to move in various directions, speeds, and complexities, enhancing

performance in sports, physical activities, and daily tasks.

- Expanding your range of motion improves balance, coordination, and agility.

4. Decreased Risk of Falls and Injuries:

- Enhanced mobility aids in fall and injury prevention, crucial for reducing disability and mortality among older adults.
- Improved balance, strength, and flexibility lower the risk of instability, tripping, and slipping, facilitating faster recovery from injuries.

5. Improved Blood Circulation:

- Good mobility contributes to cardiovascular and respiratory health, crucial components of overall well-being.
- Increased body movement elevates heart rate, blood pressure, and blood flow, delivering more oxygen and nutrients to cells and organs, thereby enhancing metabolism, immune system, and energy levels.

6. Boosted Mood and Mental Health:

- Engaging in physical activity, integral to good mobility, releases endorphins, serotonin, and dopamine, fostering a positive mood, stress reduction, and resilience against depression.

- Improved mobility positively impacts self-esteem, confidence, and social skills.

In essence, prioritizing good mobility yields multifaceted benefits, spanning the physical, mental, and emotional dimensions of well-being. Consistently working on mobility sets the stage for improved health, enhanced well-being, and increased independence, ushering in a life that is not just active but fulfilling.

What are the common causes and signs of mobility problems

Navigating Mobility Challenges: Understanding, Identifying, and Managing

Mobility problems encompass a spectrum of difficulties and limitations hindering the seamless execution of daily activities and movement. While these challenges can affect individuals of all ages, they are more prevalent among older adults and those grappling with chronic conditions or disabilities. The causes and manifestations of mobility problems are diverse, contingent upon the unique characteristics of each individual and the underlying factors at play.

Common Causes of Mobility Problems:

1. Neurological Conditions:

- Examples include stroke, Parkinson's disease, multiple sclerosis, or spinal cord injury.
- These conditions impact the brain, nerves, and muscles, leading to compromised movement, coordination, balance, and sensation.

2. Musculoskeletal Conditions:

- Conditions like arthritis, osteoporosis, or fractures fall into this category.
- Afflicting bones, joints, and muscles, these conditions induce pain, stiffness, inflammation, and weakness.

3. Cardiovascular and Respiratory Conditions:

- Heart disease, chronic obstructive pulmonary disease, or asthma are common culprits.
- Affecting the heart and lungs, they result in breathlessness, fatigue, and diminished oxygen delivery to tissues.

4. Metabolic and Endocrine Conditions:

- Diabetes, thyroid disorders, or obesity are examples in this realm.
- These conditions impact metabolism and hormones, causing weight gain, nerve damage, poor circulation, and an elevated risk of infections.

5. Mental Health Conditions:
- Depression, anxiety, or dementia contribute to mobility challenges.
- Impacting mood, cognition, and behavior, these conditions manifest as low motivation, confusion, memory loss, and a heightened fear of falling.

<u>Common Signs of Mobility Problems</u>

1. Difficulty in Movement:
- Individuals may struggle with walking, standing, or sitting, often requiring assistance or supportive devices.

2. Reduced Joint and Muscle Flexibility:
- Manifestations may include a diminished range of motion and a lack of fluidity in joint and muscle movements.

3. Poor Posture and Alignment:
- Mobility problems can lead to compromised spine and limb stability, adversely affecting posture.

4. Falls, Injuries, or Accidents:
- Recurrent falls, injuries, or accidents, or an increasing fear of falling, serve as key indicators.

5. Decreased Physical Activity and Function:

- Individuals may experience a decline in physical activity, performance, and overall functional capabilities.
- Social and recreational activities may also witness reduced participation.

The repercussions of mobility problems extend beyond the affected individual to impact the quality of life and well-being of their caregivers. Recognizing the causes and signs of these issues becomes paramount, prompting the need for timely medical and professional intervention. Proactive management not only addresses existing challenges but also mitigates the risk of further complications, fostering an environment conducive to improved mobility and enhanced overall well-being.

How to assess your mobility and set your goals

Unlocking Your Mobility Potential: A Comprehensive Guide to Assessment and Goal Setting

Mobility, the seamless ability to move your body freely across diverse situations and environments, is a cornerstone of health, well-being, and independence. Coordinated efforts from your muscles, joints, nerves, and brain culminate in the orchestration of smooth and efficient movements, empowering you to engage in daily activities, ward off injuries, and relish a high quality of life.

Embarking on a journey to assess and optimize your mobility involves a strategic approach. Here's a step-by-step guide to help you gauge your mobility and establish goals that align with your aspirations:

1. Identify Critical Mobility Areas:
- Utilize dedicated mobility assessment tools like the [Timed Up and Go Test], [30-Second Chair Stand Test], or [Berg Balance Scale].
- Measure mobility in key domains such as walking, standing, sitting, and balancing.
- Seek professional evaluation from your doctor or a physical therapist to gain valuable insights.

2. Rate Your Current Satisfaction:
- On a scale of 1 to 10, assess your satisfaction level in each mobility area.
- Document these ratings and benchmark them against normal or optimal ranges for your age and condition.

3. Reflect on Gaps and Imbalances:
- Analyze your ratings to pinpoint areas of highest and lowest satisfaction.

- Understand the interconnectedness of these areas and their collective impact on your overall well-being.
- Recognize how challenges in one domain may cascade, affecting posture, balance, and endurance.

4. Set SMART Goals:

- Craft goals that are Specific, Measurable, Achievable, Relevant, and Time-bound (SMART).
- Define what you want to achieve, determine how to measure progress, assess achievability, underscore relevance, and set a timeframe.
- **Example:** "Achieve 30 minutes of pain-free and fatigue-free walking three times a week by month-end, promoting cardiovascular health and enhancing mood."

5. Create an Action Plan and Track Progress:

- Break down each goal into manageable steps—daily, weekly, or monthly.
- Document your action plan and integrate it into your calendar.
- Regularly review and track your progress, celebrating achievements and rewarding efforts.

- In the face of obstacles or setbacks, remain resilient, adjust your plan, and glean insights from challenges.

6. Periodically Evaluate and Revise:
- Regularly assess evolving priorities, preferences, and circumstances.
- Conduct periodic evaluations, considering if goals remain relevant, realistic, and personally meaningful.
- Revisit mobility ratings, discerning improvements or declines in satisfaction levels.
- Adapt and replace goals as needed, ensuring ongoing alignment with your aspirations.

Embarking on this journey of self-assessment and goal-setting is a dynamic process, mirroring the fluidity of your mobility itself. Regular evaluations and adjustments will not only refine your goals but also fortify your commitment to nurturing and optimizing your mobility, ultimately contributing to an active and fulfilling life.

15 Mobility Exercises:

Maintaining optimal joint and muscle health is crucial for overall well-being. Incorporating mobility exercises into your routine enhances flexibility, prevents injuries, and promotes overall physical functionality. Here are fifteen indispensable mobility exercises designed to elevate your joint and muscle health:

1. Neck Rolls

- **Objective:** Enhance neck and shoulder mobility, alleviate tension, and promote better posture.

Execution:

- Stand or sit with an upright posture and relaxed shoulders.
- Gently tilt your head to the right, initiating a backward roll.
- Continue the roll to the left and then downward.
- Return your head to the starting position and repeat in the opposite direction.
- Aim for 5 to 10 neck rolls in each direction.

2. Shoulder Circles

- ✓ **Objective:** Improve shoulder mobility and flexibility while toning upper body muscles.

Execution:

- Stand with feet shoulder-width apart and arms extended horizontally.
- Cross your arms at the front and swiftly bring them backward.
- Repeat this back-and-forth movement for 30 seconds to 1 minute.
- Switch directions and repeat.

3. Arm Swings

> ✓ **Objective:** Dynamic stretching for the upper body, warming up shoulders, arms, and chest.

Execution:

- Stand with knees slightly bent, feet shoulder-width apart, and arms stretched horizontally.
- Cross your arms at the front and swiftly bring them backward.
- Repeat this dynamic movement for 30 seconds to 1 minute.

4. Chest Opener

> ✓ **Objective:** Stretch the chest and align the shoulders, promoting better posture.

Execution:

- Stand or sit tall with feet hip-width apart and arms by your sides.
- Interlace your fingers behind your back, straightening your arms.
- Lift your arms up and back, feeling a stretch in your chest and shoulders.
- Hold for 15 to 30 seconds and then release.

5. Spinal Twist

- **Objective:** Mobilize and stretch the spine, relieving lower back pain and enhancing digestion.

Execution:

- Sit on the floor with legs extended.
- Bend your right knee, crossing the foot over the left leg.
- Place the left elbow outside the right knee and the right hand on the floor behind you.
- Twist your torso to the right, looking over your right shoulder.
- Hold for 15 to 30 seconds and then switch sides.

6. Leg Circles

- **Objective:** Improve hip mobility and strengthen hip muscles.

Execution:

- Lie on your back with legs extended.
- Lift one leg and draw small circles in the air.
- Perform 10-15 circles in each direction.
- Switch legs and repeat.

7. Wrist Flexor Stretch

- **Objective:** Enhance flexibility in the wrists and forearms.

Execution:

- Extend your right arm with palm facing down.
- Use the left hand to gently press the fingers back.
- Hold for 15-30 seconds, feeling the stretch in the forearm.
- Switch arms and repeat.

8. Seated Torso Twist

- **Objective:** Mobilize the spine and improve rotational flexibility.

Execution:

- Sit cross-legged on the floor.
- Place the right hand on the left knee and the left hand behind you.
- Twist your torso to the left, looking over your left shoulder.
- Hold for 15-30 seconds and switch sides.

9. Lateral Leg Raises

- **Objective:** Target the outer hip muscles and improve leg mobility.

Execution:

- Lie on your side with legs stacked.
- Lift the top leg as high as comfortably possible.
- Lower it back down without letting it touch the bottom leg.
- Perform 10-15 repetitions on each side.

10. Calf Raises

- **Objective:** Strengthen calf muscles and improve ankle mobility.

Execution:

- Stand with feet hip-width apart.
- Rise onto the balls of your feet, lifting heels off the ground.

- Lower heels back down and repeat for 15-20 repetitions.

11. Hip Circles

- Stand with feet slightly wider than shoulder-width apart, hands on hips.
- Slowly rotate your hips, making large circles.
- Complete 10 to 20 circles in each direction.

12. Knee Hugs

- Sit on the floor, hugging your knees, and lift your feet off the ground.
- Open your arms, extend legs to a 45-degree angle, and lean back.
- Lift your torso, bend knees, and return to the starting position.
- Repeat for 10 to 20 repetitions.

13. Ankle Rolls

- Stand upright with feet hip-width apart.
- Shift weight to the right leg, pointing left toes down.
- Rotate your left foot, making small ankle circles.
- Switch sides and repeat for a full set.

14. Leg Swings

- Stand near a wall for support.

- Swing one leg forward and backward in a smooth motion.
- Gradually increase height and speed.
- Switch legs and repeat for the set.

15. Hamstring Stretch

- Sit on the floor with one leg straight and the other foot against the inner thigh.
- Extend arms forward, bending at the waist, reaching as far as possible.
- Hold for 15 to 30 seconds and switch legs.

Incorporate these exercises into your routine, gradually increasing intensity to suit your comfort level. Consistency is key to unlocking the full benefits of improved joint and muscle health, ensuring a more active and fulfilling life.

Chapter 3

Balance and Mobility Boosters

In Chapter 3, delve into the significance of balance—a crucial aspect of stability and posture. Uncover the essentials of balance, its importance, and explore practical exercises and tips for improvement. This chapter unfolds the multifaceted benefits of enhanced balance on your physical, mental, and emotional well-being, paving the way for a more active and fulfilling life.

How to combine balance and mobility exercises for greater results

Balance and mobility are foundational skills crucial for stability, fall prevention, and daily functionality. Balance involves maintaining posture and equilibrium, whether in motion or at rest, while mobility is the freedom to move effortlessly in diverse environments. The coordination of muscles, joints, nerves, strength, flexibility, and endurance is pivotal for both.

Maximizing the benefits of balance and mobility involves strategic integration in your exercise routine. Simply combining or alternating these exercises amplifies outcomes. Consider the following tips for an effective blend:

1. Diversify Target Areas: Opt for exercises that address various body parts and facets of balance and mobility. Examples include leg swings for hip mobility and balance, ankle rolls for ankle mobility and stability, and spinal twists for spinal mobility and posture.

2. Incorporate Exercise Types: Embrace a mix of static, dynamic, and functional exercises. Static exercises, like toe raises and tandem stance, enhance balance and mobility in stillness. Dynamic exercises, such as heel-to-toe walks and braiding, fortify these skills in motion. Functional exercises, like chair squats and sit-to-stand, enhance performance in daily tasks.

3. Adjust Intensity and Frequency: Tailor the intensity, duration, and frequency based on your goals, abilities, and preferences. Start with low-intensity and short-duration exercises, gradually elevating them with progress. Modify exercises by adjusting speed, adding weights, or incorporating props for increased or decreased difficulty.

4. Regularly Assess and Modify: Monitor progress using tools like stopwatches, tape measures, or balance boards. Factor in personal feedback, considering pain, fatigue, or confidence levels. Responsive modifications to exercises ensure alignment with evolving needs.

By seamlessly combining balance and mobility exercises, holistic enhancements become achievable. This integrative approach not only refines specific skills like walking, standing, and twisting but also contributes to overall health, well-being, and an enriched, active lifestyle.

How to modify and progress the exercises to suit your level and needs

15 Balance and Mobility Boosting Exercises

1. Lunge with Twist

- ✓ **Target Muscles:** Glutes, quads, hamstrings, obliques, and core.
- ✓ **Benefits:** Improves hip mobility and spinal rotation.

- Instructions:

- Stand with feet hip-width apart, holding a medicine ball or dumbbell.
- Step forward with the right foot into a lunge (both knees at 90 degrees).
- Twist torso to the right while keeping the weight close.
- Return to center and push off the right foot. Repeat on the left.
- Alternate for 10 to 15 reps per side.

2. Squat with Overhead Reach

✓ **Target Muscles:** Quads, glutes, hamstrings, calves, shoulders, and core.
✓ **Benefits:** Stretches upper back, improves posture.

- **Instructions:**
  - Stand with feet shoulder-width apart, holding dumbbells by your sides.
  - Squat down, pushing hips back and keeping chest up.
  - Stand up, pressing dumbbells overhead with arms extended.
  - Lower dumbbells to sides and repeat for 10 to 15 reps.

3. Side Lunge with Side Bend

✓ **Target Muscles:** Inner and outer thighs, glutes, obliques, and core.
✓ **Benefits:** Increases lateral range of motion, enhances flexibility.

- **Instructions:**
  - Stand with feet wider than shoulder-width apart, arms overhead.
  - Lunge to the right, bending right knee, keeping left leg straight.
  - Bend torso to the right, reaching left arm toward right foot.
  - Return to start and repeat on the other side.
  - Alternate for 10 to 15 reps per side.

4. Curtsy Lunge with Arm Sweep

✓ **Target Muscles:** Glutes, quads, hamstrings, hip abductors and adductors, shoulders.

✓ **Benefits:** Challenges balance, improves coordination.

- Instructions:

- Stand with feet hip-width apart, arms extended to the sides.
- Cross right leg behind left, lower into a curtsy lunge.
- Sweep right arm across the body, left arm behind the back.
- Stand up and switch sides, sweeping left arm across.
- Alternate for 10 to 15 reps per side.

5. Forward Lunge with Rotation

- **Target Muscles:** Glutes, quads, hamstrings, core, upper back.
- **Benefits:** Enhances hip mobility, improves spinal rotation.

- Instructions:

- Stand with feet hip-width apart, holding a medicine ball or dumbbell.
- Step forward with the right foot into a lunge.
- Rotate torso to the right, keeping the weight close.

- Return to center and push off the right foot.
- Repeat on the left, alternating for 10 to 15 reps per side.

6. Reverse Lunge with Knee Lift
- ✓ **Target Muscles:** Glutes, quads, hamstrings, hip flexors, and core.
- ✓ **Benefits:** Improves balance, stability, and lower body strength.

- Instructions:
- Stand with feet hip-width apart, hands on hips.
- Step back with the right foot into a lunge (both knees at 90 degrees).
- Drive the right knee up towards your chest as you stand.
- Step back into a lunge and repeat for 10 to 15 reps.
- Switch legs and repeat on the other side.

7. Lateral Shuffle with Tap
- ✓ **Target Muscles:** Calves, quads, hamstrings, glutes, abductors, and core.
- ✓ **Benefits:** Enhances agility, cardiovascular fitness, and lower body strength.

- Instructions:
- Stand with feet shoulder-width apart, sink into a half-squat.

- Shuffle to the right for four steps, tapping the floor with left hand.
- Shuffle to the left for four steps, tapping the floor with right hand.
- Keep chest up and core tight throughout. Repeat for 30 to 60 seconds.

8. Skater Hops

- ✓ **Target Muscles:** Glutes, quads, hamstrings, calves, abductors, and core.
- ✓ **Benefits:** Improves power, coordination, and cardiovascular fitness.

- Instructions:

- Stand with feet hip-width apart, arms by your sides.
- Hop to the right, landing on the right foot, crossing the left leg behind.
- Swing left arm across the body, right arm behind your back.
- Hop to the left, landing on the left foot, crossing the right leg behind.
- Swing right arm across the body, left arm behind your back.
- Alternate sides for 30 to 60 seconds.

9. Calf Raise with Shoulder Press

- ✓ **Target Muscles:** Calves, shoulders, and core.

✓ **Benefits:** Strengthens calves, shoulders, improves posture, and balance.

- **Instructions:**
  - Stand with feet shoulder-width apart, hold dumbbells at shoulder level.
  - Lift heels off the floor, balancing on the balls of your feet.
  - Press dumbbells overhead, extending arms fully.
  - Lower dumbbells to shoulder level and heels to the floor. Repeat for 10 to 15 reps.

10. Deadlift with Row

  - **Target Muscles:** Hamstrings, glutes, lower back, upper back, and biceps.
  - **Benefits:** Develops hamstrings, enhances hip hinge mobility, and spinal stability.

- **Instructions:**
  - Stand with feet hip-width apart, hold dumbbells in front of thighs.
  - Hinge at hips, lowering dumbbells until torso is parallel to the floor.
  - Pull dumbbells toward your chest, bending elbows, squeezing shoulder blades.
  - Lower dumbbells and extend hips to stand up. Repeat for 10 to 15 reps.

11. Single-Leg Balance with Arm Reach

- ✓ **Target Muscles:** Core, glutes, stabilizing muscles.
- ✓ **Benefits:** Enhances overall balance, stability, and core strength.

- **Instructions:**
  - Stand on your right leg, lift your left foot slightly off the ground.
  - Extend your arms forward, maintaining a straight line from head to heel.
  - Hold the position for 15 to 30 seconds.
  - Return to the starting position and switch legs.
  - Perform 3 sets on each leg.

12. Clock Reach

- ✓ **Target Muscles:** Hamstrings, quadriceps, hip flexors, and core.
- ✓ **Benefits:** Improves hip flexibility, balance, and coordination.

- **Instructions:**
  - Imagine you're at the center of a clock.
  - Stand on one leg and reach forward with the opposite hand towards 12 o'clock.
  - Return to the starting position.
  - Repeat the reach towards 3 o'clock, 6 o'clock, and 9 o'clock.
  - Perform 8-10 reaches on each leg.

13. Standing Leg Abduction

✓ **Target Muscles:** Abductors, glutes, outer thighs.

✓ **Benefits:** Strengthens hip muscles and enhances lateral stability.

- **Instructions:**
  - Stand tall, lift your right leg sideways away from your body.
  - Keep your toes pointing forward and maintain a straight posture.
  - Hold for a moment, then lower the leg.
  - Repeat on the other leg.
  - Perform 12-15 repetitions on each leg.

14. Stability Ball Knee Tuck

✓ **Target Muscles:** Core, hip flexors, shoulders.

✓ **Benefits:** Challenges core stability and enhances overall balance.

- **Instructions:**
  - Start in a plank position with your feet on a stability ball.
  - Engage your core and bring your knees towards your chest.
  - Roll the stability ball back to the starting position.
  - Perform 10-12 repetitions.

15. Dynamic Balance Drill

- **Target Muscles:** Quads, hamstrings, calves, stabilizing muscles.
- **Benefits:** Enhances dynamic balance, coordination, and agility.

- Instructions:

- Set up cones or markers in a straight line.
- Stand on one leg and hop over each cone, maintaining balance.
- Continue hopping back and forth along the line.
- Perform for 1-2 minutes.
- Challenge yourself by increasing speed or adding more cones.

Perform these exercises as a circuit or incorporate them into your regular workout routine to enhance balance, mobility, and overall fitness. Remember to warm up and cool down for a comprehensive workout experience. Enjoy the challenge and the numerous benefits! Always prioritize proper form and gradually increase difficulty to ensure a safe and effective workout.

Chapter 4

Balance and Mobility Challenges

Delve into the crucial aspects of maintaining stability and free movement. Explore the causes and signs of balance and mobility issues, assess your current status, and set effective goals. Learn to adapt and advance exercises based on your needs and seamlessly integrate them into your daily routine. Empower yourself to conquer challenges and embrace a more active and fulfilling life.

How to Challenge your Balance and Mobility with Different Equipment, Surfaces, and Movements

Enhancing your balance and mobility is crucial for preventing falls, boosting performance, and elevating your overall well-being. Age, injury, or illness can impact these abilities, affecting your independence and quality of life. To effectively improve balance and mobility, incorporating diverse exercises is key. Repeating the same routines may lead to stagnation, hindering progress. Thus, it's vital to introduce variety by leveraging different equipment, surfaces, and movements. Here's a guide on how to achieve this:

1. Utilize Varied Equipment:

- Integrate household items like chairs, pillows, towels, or books.
- Consider fitness tools such as dumbbells, resistance bands, balance boards, or foam rollers.
- **Example:** Perform squats holding dumbbells, enhance stability with a balance board during shoulder presses, or incorporate a foam roller into leg lifts.

2. Experiment with Different Surfaces:

- Opt for surfaces like the floor, mats, carpets, beds, couches, benches, or steps.
- **Example:** Execute lunges on a carpet, engage in bed-based sit-ups, perform push-ups on a couch, practice dips using a bench, or elevate your routine with step-ups on a step.

3. Embrace Diverse Movements:

- Challenge coordination, agility, and flexibility by incorporating varied directions, speeds, and complexities.
- **Example:** Walk forward, backward, sideways, or diagonally; alter running speeds or intervals; introduce diverse jumping patterns.

By infusing your routine with diverse equipment, surfaces, and movements, you infuse an element of enjoyment and effectiveness into your balance and mobility training. This not only aids in improving these skills but also contributes to overall health, well-being, and independence, paving the way for a more active and fulfilling life.

How to Add Variety and Fun to your Balance and Mobility Exercises

Elevating your stability and flexibility through balance and mobility exercises is a crucial aspect of overall well-being. While these exercises are instrumental in preventing falls and enhancing performance, the repetitive nature of the same routines can lead to boredom and diminished effectiveness. To ensure continuous improvement, injecting variety and enjoyment into your regimen is essential. Here's a comprehensive guide on how to achieve this:

1. Diversify Equipment Usage:

- Incorporate household items like chairs, pillows, towels, or books.
- Explore fitness equipment such as dumbbells, resistance bands, balance boards, or foam rollers.
- **Example:** Engage in squats with dumbbells, introduce stability with a balance board during

shoulder presses, or enhance flexibility using a foam roller during leg lifts.

2. Explore Different Surfaces:

- Utilize various surfaces like the floor, mats, carpets, beds, couches, benches, or steps.
- **Example:** Execute lunges on a carpet, perform sit-ups on a bed, engage in push-ups on a couch, try dips on a bench, or add complexity with step-ups on a step.

3. Incorporate Varied Movements:

- Challenge coordination, agility, and flexibility with diverse directions, speeds, and complexities.
- **Example:** Experiment with walking forward, backward, sideways, or diagonally; vary running speeds or intervals; introduce dynamic jumping patterns.

4. Infuse Fun Elements:

- Incorporate games, or challenges to make your exercises more enjoyable and motivational.
- Listen to favorite songs, podcasts, or audiobooks during exercises or create playlists matching your workout's tempo and mood.

- Engage in games like Simon Says, Twister, or Hopscotch that integrate balance and mobility skills.
- Challenge yourself, friends, family, or online community to meet specific exercise goals or attempt new and challenging variations.

By infusing variety and fun into your balance and mobility exercises, you not only enhance their effectiveness but also make the journey to improved stability and flexibility more enjoyable. This holistic approach contributes not only to physical health but also overall well-being, fostering a more active and fulfilling life.

How to prevent and overcome common balance and mobility issues

Maintaining stability and the ability to move freely are crucial for overall well-being, particularly in preventing falls and enhancing daily performance. However, factors such as age, injury, or illness can impact balance and mobility, affecting independence and quality of life. To address and overcome common challenges, consider the following comprehensive tips:

1. Incorporate Regular Exercise:

- Engage in exercises targeting strength, flexibility, endurance, and coordination.
- Include balance-enhancing activities like lunges, squats, leg swings, or heel-to-toe walks.
- Prioritize at least 150 minutes of moderate-intensity physical activity weekly, adjusting as per medical recommendations.

2. Assess Medications and Supplements:

- Evaluate medications and supplements for potential side effects impacting balance.
- Consult with healthcare professionals to adjust dosage, timing, or type if necessary.
- Avoid substances, including alcohol that may contribute to drowsiness, dizziness, or low blood pressure.

3. Manage Health Conditions:

- Address underlying health conditions like diabetes, arthritis, osteoporosis, or Parkinson's disease.
- Follow medical advice for controlling blood sugar, reducing inflammation, preventing bone loss, or managing movement disorders.

- Seek prompt medical attention for any new or worsening symptoms, such as pain, numbness, tingling, or tremors.

4. Prioritize Vision and Hearing Health:

- Regularly check and maintain vision and hearing aids, if prescribed.
- Avoid environmental factors that may impair vision or hearing, such as dim lighting or loud noises.
- Consult with eye or ear specialists promptly if issues arise.

5. Create a Safe Environment:

- Modify home and work environments to enhance safety and comfort.
- Remove potential hazards like clutter, cords, rugs, or obstacles that could lead to tripping or slipping.
- Install grab bars, handrails, or ramps as needed and use nonskid mats, rubber-soled shoes, or assistive devices to prevent falls.
- Adjust lighting, temperature, and furniture to suit personal needs.

By adhering to these comprehensive tips, you will proactively prevent and overcome common balance and mobility issues, thereby enhancing their overall quality of life and preserving independence. Always consult with a healthcare professional before embarking on new exercises or medications, and seek assistance when concerns or questions arise. With proper care and attention, maintaining or improving balance and mobility becomes an achievable goal, leading to a more active and fulfilling life.

15 Balance and Mobility Challenges:

1. BOSU Ball Squat
2. Stability Ball Bridge
3. Foam Roller Plank
4. Resistance Band Row
5. Medicine Ball Slam
6. Kettlebell Swing
7. TRX Suspension Trainer Squat
8. Agility Ladder Run
9. Balance Board Twist
10. Wobble Cushion Stand
11. Box Jump
12. Bosu Ball Plank
13. Cone Shuffles
14. Dumbbell Single-Leg Romanian Deadlift
15. Jumping Lunges

<u>Balance and Mobility Challenges</u>

Balance and mobility are indispensable skills that contribute to our daily life and athletic achievements, promoting stability, fall prevention, and efficient movement. To further enhance these skills, engaging in specific challenges can provide a multifaceted approach, addressing strength, endurance, coordination, and flexibility. Here, we present 15 diverse balance and mobility challenges suitable for home or gym settings, utilizing equipment such as BOSU balls, stability balls, foam rollers, resistance bands, medicine balls, kettlebells, TRX suspension trainers, agility ladders, balance boards, and wobble cushions. These challenges cater to various fitness levels and offer the flexibility to modify or progress based on individual needs.

Before You Begin:
- ✓ Ensure a proper warm-up routine and adequate safety measures.
- ✓ Consult with a doctor or physical therapist if you have medical conditions or injuries.

1. BOSU Ball Squat
- ✓ **Equipment Needed:** BOSU ball (flat or curved side up based on preference).

Execution:
- Stand on the BOSU ball with feet shoulder-width apart.
- Extend arms for balance, keeping chest up and core engaged.

- Hinge at hips, bend knees into a squat position.
- Push through heels, squeezing glutes, and return to the starting position.

2. Stability Ball Bridge
✓ **Equipment Needed:** Stability ball.

Execution:

- Lie on your back with feet on the stability ball.
- Press shoulders into the floor, lifting hips until a straight line forms.
- Hold briefly, then lower hips back to the floor.

3. Foam Roller Plank
✓ **Equipment Needed:** Foam roller.

Execution:

- Get into a plank position with hands on the foam roller.
- Maintain a straight line from head to heels.
- Hold position or add difficulty by rolling the foam roller slightly.

4. Resistance Band Row
✓ **Equipment Needed:** Resistance band.

Execution:

- Anchor the band securely and stand facing the anchor.
- Hinge at hips, keeping back straight.

- Pull the band towards your chest, squeezing shoulder blades together.
- Slowly extend arms and return to starting position.

5. Medicine Ball Slam

✓ **Equipment Needed:** Medicine ball.

Execution:

- Stand with feet shoulder-width apart, holding the medicine ball.
- Lift the ball overhead, slam it onto the floor.
- Bend knees and hips, catch the ball, and repeat.

These challenges encompass a range of movements targeting various muscle groups and aspects of balance and mobility. Integrate them into your routine, adjusting intensity and repetitions as needed. As you progress, not only will you notice improvements in stability and mobility, but you'll also enjoy the added benefits of enhanced strength, coordination, and cardiovascular fitness.

6. Kettlebell Swing

The kettlebell swing is a dynamic exercise that targets explosive power, strength, speed, and cardiovascular fitness. Proper execution is crucial for maximizing benefits and minimizing the risk of injury.

Equipment Needed:

✓ Kettlebell (weight depends on fitness level)

Execution:

1. Setup:

- Place the kettlebell on the floor, slightly wider than hip-distance apart.
- Stand with feet shoulder-width apart, toes angled out slightly.

2. Initial Position:

- Hinge at the hips, bending knees slightly to grasp the kettlebell handle with both hands.
- Maintain a straight back, chest up, and engage the core.

3. Swinging Motion:

- Swing the kettlebell back between your legs, keeping arms straight and shoulders relaxed.
- In one explosive movement, squeeze glutes and thrust hips forward to swing the kettlebell up to chest level.
- Keep arms straight and core tight, avoiding arching the back or neck.

4. Downward Swing

- Allow the kettlebell to swing back down between your legs as you hinge at the hips and bend knees slightly.

5. Repetition:

- Repeat the swinging motion for the desired number of reps or time.

7. TRX Suspension Trainer Squat

The TRX suspension trainer squat is an effective lower body exercise that challenges quads, glutes, and calves, while also engaging core stability and ankle mobility.

Equipment Needed:
- TRX Suspension Trainer

Execution:
1. Setup:
- Attach the TRX suspension trainer to a secure anchor point, adjusting straps to a medium length.
- Stand facing the anchor point with feet shoulder-width apart, toes pointing forward.

2. Initial Position:
- Hold TRX handles with palms facing each other, arms extended in front.
- Keep shoulders down, back straight, and core engaged.

3. Squatting Motion:
- Lean back slightly and bend knees to lower into a squat position.

- Ensure weight is on heels, and knees align with toes. Avoid knees collapsing or chest dropping.

4. Return to Starting Position:
- Push through heels, squeezing glutes, to return to the starting position.

5. Repetition:
- Repeat the squatting motion for the desired number of reps or time.

8. Agility Ladder Run

The agility ladder run is a dynamic exercise focusing on footwork, agility, speed, and cardiovascular fitness.

Equipment Needed:
  ✓ Agility ladder

Execution:
1. Setup:
  - Place the agility ladder on the floor.

2. Starting Position:
- Stand at one end of the ladder with feet together, toes pointing forward.

3. Running Through the Ladder
- Run through the ladder, placing one foot in each rung as fast as possible.

- Pump arms and lift knees high, avoiding touching rungs or ladder edges.

4. Direction Change:
- Upon reaching the end, turn around and run back through the ladder in the opposite direction.

5. Repetition:
- Repeat the running motion through the ladder for the desired number of reps or time.

9. Balance Board Twist

The balance board twist is an effective exercise targeting core, obliques, and lower back, while improving balance and posture.

Equipment Needed:
- ✓ Balance board

Execution:

1. Setup:
- Place the balance board on the floor.

2. Starting Position:
- Stand on the balance board with feet hip-width apart, toes pointing forward.

3. Twisting Motion:

- Extend arms to the sides at shoulder level, keeping chest up, shoulders back, and core engaged.
- Twist torso to the right, rotating the balance board as far as possible while maintaining hip and leg stability.
- Return to center and then twist to the left, repeating the twisting motion.

4. Repetition:
- Repeat the twisting motion from side to side for the desired number of reps or time.

10. Wobble Cushion Stand

The wobble cushion stand is a challenging exercise that strengthens lower leg muscles, specifically the peroneals, and enhances overall balance and coordination.

Equipment Needed:
- ✓ Wobble cushion

Execution:

1. Setup:
- Place the wobble cushion on the floor.

2. Starting Position:
- Stand on the wobble cushion with feet together, toes pointing forward.

3. Stability:

- Keep knees slightly bent, back straight, and engage the core.
- Press shoulders into the floor for added stability.

4. Balance Challenge:

- Hold this position for the desired amount of time.
- To increase difficulty, lift one foot off the cushion, close your eyes, or add arm movements.

11. Box Jump

The box jump is a plyometric exercise that enhances explosive power, strength, and coordination while challenging your balance.

Equipment Needed:

✓ Sturdy box or platform

Execution:

1. Setup:

- Place a sturdy box or platform in front of you.

2. Starting Position:

- Stand with feet shoulder-width apart, toes pointing forward.

3. Jumping Motion:

- Bend at the knees and hips, swinging arms back.
- Explosively jump onto the box, extending hips and knees fully.

4. Landing:

- Land softly on the box, ensuring proper alignment of knees and ankles.
- Stand upright on the box.

5. Step Down:

- Step back down to the starting position.

6. Repetition:

- Repeat the jumping motion for the desired number of reps or time.

12. Bosu Ball Plank

The Bosu ball plank challenges core stability, shoulder strength, and overall balance, providing a dynamic twist to the traditional plank.

Equipment Needed:
  ✓ Bosu ball

Execution:
  1. Setup:

- Place the Bosu ball on the floor with the dome side down.

2. Planking Position:

- Assume a plank position with hands on the flat side of the Bosu ball, shoulders directly above wrists.

3. Core Engagement:

- Engage the core, ensuring a straight line from head to heels.

4. Hold:

- Maintain the plank position for the desired amount of time.

5. Variation:

- To increase difficulty, lift one arm or leg off the Bosu ball.

6. Repetition:

- Repeat the exercise for the desired number of reps or time.

13. Cone Shuffles

Cone shuffles improve lateral movement, agility, and coordination, providing a dynamic challenge to your balance and mobility.

Equipment Needed:
- ✓ Cones or markers

Execution:

1. Setup:
- Place cones or markers in a straight line, with ample space between each.

2. Starting Position:
- Stand next to the first cone with feet together.

3. Shuffling Motion:
- Shuffle laterally to the next cone, keeping feet close to the ground.

4. Quick Feet:
- Perform quick, controlled steps, emphasizing agility and balance.

5. Touch and Go:
- Touch the cone with one hand before shuffling back to the starting position.

6. Repeat:
- Repeat the shuffling motion to the next cone and back for the desired number of reps.

14. Dumbbell Single-Leg Romanian Deadlift

This exercise targets the hamstrings, glutes, and lower back while challenging balance and stability.

Equipment Needed:
- ✓ Dumbbells

Execution:

1. Setup:
- Hold a dumbbell in each hand with feet hip-width apart.

2. Single-Leg Stance:
- Shift weight onto one leg, keeping a slight bend in the knee.

3. Hinging Forward:
- Hinge at the hips, extending the free leg straight behind.

4. Maintain Alignment:
- Keep the back straight, and extend the dumbbells toward the floor.

5. Return to Upright Position:
- Engage the glutes and hamstrings to return to an upright position.

6. Repeat:

- Perform the movement on one leg for the desired number of reps before switching legs.

15. Jumping Lunges

Jumping lunges add an explosive element to traditional lunges, targeting the quads, hamstrings, and glutes while improving balance and coordination.

Equipment Needed:
- ✓ None (bodyweight exercise)

Execution:

1. Starting Position:
- Stand with feet together.

2. Lunge Position:
- Take a step forward with the right foot, bending both knees to 90 degrees.

3. Jumping Motion:
- Explosively jump into the air, switching the position of the feet mid-air.

4. Landing:
- Land softly in a lunge position with the left foot forward.

5. Repeat:

- Jump back and forth, alternating legs, for the desired number of reps or time.

By incorporating these challenging yet effective exercises into your routine, you can elevate your balance, mobility, and overall fitness. Always prioritize proper form and safety precautions to maximize the benefits of these movements.

10 additional exercises to further enhance balance and mobility

1.   Single-Leg RDL (Romanian Deadlift)
Equipment Needed: Dumbbells or Kettlebells
Instructions:
- Stand on one leg with a slight bend in the knee.
- Hold a dumbbell or kettlebell in one or both hands in front of you.
- Hinge at your hips, lowering the weight toward the ground while extending your free leg straight behind you.
- Keep your back straight and chest up throughout the movement.
- Return to the starting position and repeat for 12 reps on each leg.

2. Side Plank with Leg Lift
Equipment Needed: Exercise Mat
Instructions:
- Begin in a side plank position on your elbow, with your body in a straight line.
- Lift your top leg upward while keeping your core engaged and hips stable.
- Lower the leg back down and repeat for 12 reps on each side.
- Focus on maintaining proper form and control throughout the exercise.

3. Clock Lunges

Equipment Needed: None

Instructions:

- Stand with your feet together as if you were at the center of a clock.
- Step forward to 12 o'clock with your right foot, then return to the center.
- Repeat the lunge to 1 o'clock, then back to the center, and continue in a clockwise direction.
- Perform lunges in each direction, then switch to counterclockwise.
- Aim for 12 lunges in each direction.

4. Plank with Shoulder Taps

Equipment Needed: Exercise Mat

Instructions:

- Start in a plank position with your hands directly under your shoulders.
- Lift one hand and tap the opposite shoulder while keeping your hips stable.
- Return the hand to the floor and repeat on the other side.
- Maintain a straight line from head to heels throughout the exercise.
- Perform 15 taps on each shoulder.

5. Step-Ups with Knee Drive

Equipment Needed: Step or Bench

Instructions:

- Stand in front of a step or bench.
- Step up with your right foot, driving your left knee toward your chest.
- Lower your left foot back down and switch to the left foot stepping up.
- Continue alternating legs and add a knee drive with each step-up.
- Perform 15 step-ups on each leg.

6. Side Plank with Rotation

Equipment Needed: Exercise Mat

Instructions:

- Begin in a side plank position on your elbow, with your body forming a straight line.
- Rotate your torso, bringing your free arm underneath your body and reaching towards the floor.
- Return to the starting side plank position and repeat the rotation.
- Perform 12 rotations on each side, focusing on controlled movements.

7. Jumping Lunges

Equipment Needed: None

Instructions:

- Start in a lunge position with your right foot forward and left foot back.
- Jump explosively, switching your leg positions mid-air.
- Land softly in a lunge with your left foot forward.
- Continue jumping and alternating legs for a total of 20 lunges (10 on each leg).

8. Plank to Downward Dog

Equipment Needed: Exercise Mat

Instructions:

- Begin in a plank position with your hands directly under your shoulders.
- Lift your hips towards the ceiling, moving into a downward dog position.
- Hold for a moment, feeling the stretch in your hamstrings and calves.
- Return to the plank position and repeat for 15 repetitions.

9. Lateral Band Walk

Equipment Needed: Resistance Band

Instructions:

- Place a resistance band around your legs, just above the knees.
- Stand with your feet hip-width apart and a slight bend in your knees.

- Take a step to the right, maintaining tension in the band, then follow with your left foot.
- Perform 15 steps to the right and then 15 steps to the left.

10. Single-Leg Balance with Reach

Equipment Needed: None

Instructions:

- Stand on your right leg with a slight bend in the knee.
- Extend your left leg behind you, keeping it in line with your body.
- Reach your left hand towards the floor while extending your right arm forward.
- Return to the starting position and repeat for 12 repetitions on each leg.

These exercises add variety and complexity to your balance and mobility routine, engaging different muscle groups and challenging your coordination. Remember to start with an appropriate level of difficulty and gradually progress as you feel more confident and comfortable with each movement.

Conclusion

In concluding this comprehensive guide, "Fast and Effective Exercises for Seniors: 60 Moves to Boost Balance and Mobility," I want to express my heartfelt gratitude for embarking on this transformative journey with me. Your commitment to enhancing your well-being and embracing a more active lifestyle is truly commendable.

As we conclude this empowering exploration, I encourage you to reflect on the progress you've made, the newfound strength you've discovered, and the improved balance and mobility that now define your daily life. This book was crafted with your needs in mind, aiming to provide a holistic approach to senior fitness that goes beyond mere exercises—it's a testament to the vitality and resilience within you.

Your decision to invest in this guide was a pledge to prioritize your health, and for that, I applaud you. Now equipped with a repertoire of 60 exercises tailored for seniors, each move has been carefully curated to address the unique requirements of your body, fostering balance, mobility, and overall vitality.

As you incorporate these exercises into your routine, remember the **"why"** that led you to this book—the desire for a more fulfilling and active life. Embrace the sense of accomplishment with each completed workout and celebrate the small victories that pave the way for significant transformations.

I invite you to share your experiences and insights by leaving a review. Your feedback is invaluable—it not only encourages others to embark on this journey but also contributes to the collective spirit of support within our community.

Thank you for choosing **"Fast and Effective Exercises for Seniors."** May your newfound strength be a source of inspiration, and may your journey continue to unfold with vitality, balance, and enduring well-being.

Wishing you a life filled with health, happiness, and the joy of movement.

With gratitude,

[Body Walker]

Bonus

30-Day Senior Fitness Challenge

Boosting Balance and Mobility

Weeks 1-2: Establishing Foundation

Day 1-3:

1. **BOSU Ball Squat:** 3 sets of 10 reps
2. **Stability Ball Bridge:** 3 sets of 12 reps
3. **Foam Roller Plank:** 3 sets, hold for 30 seconds each

Day 4-7:

4. Resistance Band Row: 3 sets of 12 reps
5. Medicine Ball Slam: 3 sets of 10 reps
6. Kettlebell Swing: 3 sets of 10 reps

Weeks 3-4: Building Endurance

Day 8-10:

7. **TRX Suspension Trainer Squat:** 3 sets of 12 reps
8. **Agility Ladder Run:** 3 sets, 1 minute each
9. **Balance Board Twist:** 3 sets of 12 reps per side

Day 11-14:

10. **Wobble Cushion Stand:** 3 sets, hold for 45 seconds
11. **Reverse Lunge with Knee Lift:** 3 sets of 12 reps per leg
12. **Lateral Shuffle with Tap:** 3 sets, 45 seconds each side

Weeks 5-6: Adding Complexity

Day 15-17:

13. **Calf Raise with Shoulder Press:** 3 sets of 15 reps
14. **Deadlift with Row:** 3 sets of 12 reps
15. **Forward Lunge with Rotation:** 3 sets of 12 reps per side

Day 18-21:

16. **Skater Hops:** 3 sets, 1 minute
17. **Curtsy Lunge with Arm Sweep:** 3 sets of 12 reps per side
18. **Lunge with Twist:** 3 sets of 12 reps per side

Weeks 7-8: Intensifying the Challenge

Day 22-24:

19. **Reverse Lunge with Knee Lift:** 3 sets of 12 reps per leg
20. **Lateral Shuffle with Tap:** 3 sets, 1 minute
21. **Skater Hops:** 3 sets, 1 minute

Day 25-28:

22. **Calf Raise with Shoulder Press:** 3 sets of 15 reps
23. **Deadlift with Row:** 3 sets of 12 reps
24. **Forward Lunge with Rotation:** 3 sets of 12 reps per side

Weeks 9-10: Mastering Mobility

Day 29-30:

25. **Skater Hops:** 4 sets, 1 minute
26. **Lateral Shuffle with Tap:** 4 sets, 1 minute
27. **Deadlift with Row:** 4 sets of 12 reps

Celebrate your progress, and feel free to modify exercises based on your comfort level. Always consult with your healthcare provider before starting a new workout routine. Enjoy the journey to improved balance and mobility!

Glossary of Terms

1. Antihypertensives:

Medications that help lower high blood pressure.

2. Sarcopenia:

Age-related loss of muscle mass and strength.

3. Presbycusis:

Age-related hearing loss.

4. Tibialis Anterior:

The muscle that helps lift the front of your foot.

5. Pilates:

A low-impact exercise method emphasizing flexibility, core strength, and body awareness.

Index